Low-FODMAP Meal Plan

Delicious, Digestive-Friendly Meals for
IBS Relief

Sasha Ramsay A.

Table of contents

Introduction

When you embark on a journey to improve your well-being, the food on your plate becomes your greatest ally or your worst enemy. For those dealing with the discomfort and unpredictability of IBS, this couldn't be more true. But imagine waking up each day, enjoying meals without second-guessing whether they'll leave you bloated, cramping, or running for the bathroom. What if the joy of eating could return—without the constant fear of triggering symptoms that drain your energy and make social gatherings feel like a gamble? This is what the Low-FODMAP diet promises. It's not a restriction, but rather a gateway to relief and vitality.

In a world of endless diet plans and fads, the Low-FODMAP diet stands out because it's backed by science and tailored specifically for those like you, searching for a real solution to manage IBS. This is not just about cutting out foods; it's about rediscovering your relationship with what you eat. It's about understanding your body and finally regaining control over your digestive health. Imagine the freedom of knowing exactly what fuels your body without any unwanted surprises—this book will be your trusted guide to that freedom.

Whether you're completely new to the Low-FODMAP lifestyle or you've tried it before and felt lost in a maze of labels and lists, you're about to embark on an empowering journey. Here, you'll find not only practical advice but also delicious meals that nurture both your gut and your taste buds. This is about taking back the joy of eating—bite by bite. It's about turning the kitchen from a place of stress into a sanctuary of flavor, comfort, and, most importantly, relief.

This book is your road map to a lifestyle that is achievable, sustainable, and utterly delicious. Each recipe has been thoughtfully crafted not just to keep your IBS in check but to bring you the joy of truly enjoying food again. No more feeling like you're missing out. No more bland meals or endless internet searches for what you "can" or "can't" eat. With the tips and recipes you'll find within these pages, you'll experience the satisfaction of knowing that every ingredient has been carefully chosen to keep your digestion in harmony.

As you turn each page, let your excitement grow—because the recipes waiting for you aren't just meals, they're the key to living symptom-free. You won't be staring at a diet that feels like deprivation but rather embracing a lifestyle that enhances your daily life. This is your chance to break free from the chains of IBS, armed with the knowledge and the tools to make every meal a celebration, not a cause for concern.

Let's transform your kitchen, your diet, and most importantly, your relationship with food. This book is more than just recipes; it's a path toward relief, vitality, and a brighter, symptom-free tomorrow.

Chapter 1: Understanding the Low-FODMAP Diet

What are FODMAPs?

FODMAPs, short for fermentable oligosaccharides, disaccharides, monosaccharides, and polyols, are specific types of carbohydrates that some people struggle to digest properly. These are naturally found in a wide variety of foods, and while they don't cause issues for most, individuals with Irritable Bowel Syndrome (IBS) often find that these compounds trigger uncomfortable and sometimes debilitating digestive symptoms. But what exactly do these scientific-sounding terms mean?

Let's break it down: Oligosaccharides are found in foods like wheat, garlic, onions, and legumes. Disaccharides include lactose, which is present in dairy products like milk and yogurt. Monosaccharides are primarily found in foods rich in fructose, such as certain fruits, honey, and sweeteners like high-fructose corn syrup. Lastly, polyols are sugar alcohols present in foods such as apples, cauliflower, and artificial sweeteners like sorbitol and xylitol.

When you consume foods high in FODMAPs, they aren't fully absorbed in the small intestine, leading to fermentation in the colon. This process can cause gas, bloating, and changes in bowel habits, including diarrhea and constipation—all hallmark symptoms of IBS. Since these carbohydrates draw water into the intestines, they can also lead to discomfort, stomach distension, and other IBS-related issues.

For many people, simply knowing that certain foods contain FODMAPs and understanding how they affect the digestive system can be an "aha" moment. It's not about a lack of willpower or sensitivity; it's about the unique way your body processes certain carbohydrates. By becoming aware of what FODMAPs are and how they behave in the gut, you're taking the first empowering step towards managing your IBS and regaining control over your digestive health.

How the Low-FODMAP Diet Helps with IBS

The Low-FODMAP diet is not just another restrictive eating plan; it is a scientifically-backed approach designed to help those with IBS minimize their symptoms. Research conducted by Monash University in Australia has shown that reducing the intake of FODMAPs can significantly reduce IBS symptoms in the majority of sufferers. This diet is not about eliminating all types of carbohydrates—rather, it focuses on limiting those that are poorly absorbed by the gut.

By reducing the amount of FODMAPs you consume, you're essentially reducing the amount of fermentation that takes place in your digestive system. This lowers the production of gas, reduces bloating, and helps regulate your bowel movements, providing relief from both constipation and diarrhea. In short, the Low-FODMAP diet can help create a calmer, more predictable digestive experience.

But what makes this diet so powerful for managing IBS isn't just the short-term relief it provides. The long-term benefits lie in its personalized approach. Once you've reduced your intake of FODMAPs and experienced symptom relief, the next step is to gradually reintroduce foods to pinpoint your unique triggers. This gives you the tools to not only avoid discomfort but also to enjoy a wider variety of foods without fear. The Low-FODMAP diet teaches you how to listen to your body, understand its signals, and make informed choices that support your digestive health.

For many IBS sufferers, the Low-FODMAP diet can feel like unlocking the secret to a life that isn't dictated by the whims of their digestive system. The goal isn't just symptom relief—it's empowerment and the ability to enjoy food and life again without the constant worry of discomfort or embarrassment.

Introduction to the Phases: Elimination and Reintroduction

The Low-FODMAP diet is structured into two key phases: the Elimination phase and the Reintroduction phase. Each plays a vital role in helping you understand which specific foods trigger your IBS symptoms, providing long-term relief while allowing for greater dietary flexibility.

The **Elimination Phase** is the first step and typically lasts between four to six weeks. During this time, you'll strictly limit your intake of high-FODMAP foods. While this might sound restrictive, it's important to focus on the many delicious, Low-FODMAP alternatives that are available. This phase is critical because it gives your digestive system time to reset, allowing you to experience significant symptom relief. For many people, the Elimination phase can be life-changing, as it provides a clear contrast between the chaos of unpredictable IBS symptoms and the calm that comes from managing them through diet.

After you've completed the Elimination phase and experienced relief, the **Reintroduction Phase** begins. This is where the magic of personalization happens. During this phase, you'll slowly reintroduce high-FODMAP foods one at a time, carefully monitoring your symptoms to identify which foods trigger discomfort. The reintroduction process is methodical, and it requires patience, but the insights you gain are invaluable.

Through this phase, you'll discover which specific FODMAPs your body can tolerate and which ones you should avoid. This is key because everyone's triggers are different. While one person might be able to tolerate lactose, another may find that fructose is their main issue. The Reintroduction phase allows you to create a personalized roadmap for your diet, where you can confidently enjoy a wide variety of foods without fear of triggering symptoms.

The combination of the Elimination and Reintroduction phases gives you a deeper understanding of your body and its needs, ultimately leading to a sustainable way of eating that's not just about avoiding discomfort but also about reclaiming the joy of eating.

Navigating Grocery Shopping on a Low-FODMAP Diet

One of the biggest challenges people face when starting a Low-FODMAP diet is grocery shopping. Suddenly, ingredients that you once thought were harmless could now trigger your symptoms. But don't worry—grocery shopping on a Low-FODMAP diet doesn't have to be overwhelming once you know what to look for and how to plan ahead.

First, it's crucial to become familiar with the foods that are naturally Low-FODMAP. Fresh produce like carrots, zucchini, spinach, and potatoes are your best friends. Proteins such as eggs, chicken, turkey, and fish are also safe bets. Dairy can be tricky, but opting for lactose-free versions of milk, cheese, and yogurt will help keep symptoms at bay. For grains, look for gluten-free products, as many regular wheat-based items are high in FODMAPs.

When shopping for packaged foods, always check labels carefully. Many processed items contain hidden FODMAPs like high-fructose corn syrup, inulin, or artificial sweeteners. Stick to brands that you trust, or better yet, try to stick to whole, unprocessed foods as much as possible.

Meal planning is also key to successful Low-FODMAP grocery shopping. Before you head to the store, it's helpful to have a plan for the week's meals. This not only saves time but also ensures that you don't accidentally buy ingredients that could trigger symptoms. Armed with a list of Low-FODMAP foods, grocery shopping becomes less of a daunting task and more of an opportunity to discover new, gut-friendly foods and flavors.

Over time, navigating the grocery store will become second nature, and you'll build a repertoire of trusted brands and products. With a little preparation, you can turn shopping into an experience that supports your Low-FODMAP lifestyle while keeping your meals exciting and varied.

Tips for a Smooth Transition

Transitioning to a Low-FODMAP diet can feel overwhelming at first, but with the right approach, it can be a seamless and positive change. One of the most important things to remember is that this is a journey, not an overnight transformation. Give yourself grace, and focus on the small, achievable steps that will help you succeed.

Start by educating yourself. Knowledge is power when it comes to managing IBS through diet. Familiarize yourself with which foods are Low-FODMAP and which ones should be avoided. Don't hesitate to keep a list or download a Low-FODMAP app to help you navigate choices in real-time, especially when eating out or trying new recipes.

Another key tip is to plan your meals in advance. Knowing what you'll be eating for the week removes the stress of last-minute decisions that could lead to consuming a high-FODMAP food by mistake. Batch cooking and meal prepping will also help you stick to the plan when life gets busy.

Additionally, don't be afraid to experiment in the kitchen. One of the misconceptions about the Low-FODMAP diet is that it's restrictive, but the reality is that there are plenty of delicious foods and recipes to explore. Try new ingredients and keep your meals varied to prevent boredom and ensure that you're getting a wide range of nutrients.

Lastly, listen to your body and be patient with yourself. Your digestive system needs time to adjust, and results won't happen overnight. But with persistence and the right mindset, the transition will become easier, and before you know it, you'll be enjoying the benefits of a Low-FODMAP lifestyle, symptom-free and feeling empowered.

Chapter 2: Breakfasts to Start the Day Right

Low-FODMAP Banana Oat Pancakes

Ingredients:

- 1 ripe banana
- 1 cup gluten-free oats
- 1/2 cup lactose-free milk or almond milk
- 1 egg
- 1 tsp vanilla extract
- 1/2 tsp cinnamon
- 1 tsp baking powder
- A pinch of salt
- 1 tbsp maple syrup (optional)
- Coconut oil for cooking

Cooking Instructions:

1. In a blender, combine the banana, oats, milk, egg, vanilla extract, cinnamon, baking powder, and salt. Blend until smooth.
2. Heat a non-stick skillet over medium heat and lightly grease with coconut oil.
3. Pour small amounts of batter (about 1/4 cup per pancake) into the skillet and cook for 2-3 minutes on each side, until golden brown.
4. Serve warm with a drizzle of maple syrup or Low-FODMAP fruits like strawberries or blueberries.

Cook Tips:

- For extra fluffiness, let the batter rest for 5 minutes before cooking.
- You can also fold in blueberries or chocolate chips for added flavor.

Nutritional Value (per serving):

- Calories: 250
- Protein: 8g
- Carbohydrates: 45g
- Fat: 6g
- Fiber: 4g

Chia Pudding with Blueberries

Ingredients:

- 1/4 cup chia seeds
- 1 cup lactose-free milk or almond milk
- 1 tsp vanilla extract
- 1 tbsp maple syrup or stevia (optional)
- 1/4 cup fresh blueberries

Cooking Instructions:

1. In a bowl, whisk together the chia seeds, milk, vanilla extract, and maple syrup.
2. Let the mixture sit for 5 minutes, then whisk again to prevent clumping.
3. Cover and refrigerate for at least 2 hours or overnight until it thickens into a pudding-like consistency.
4. Serve with fresh blueberries on top.

Cook Tips:

- For a creamier texture, blend the chia seed mixture before refrigerating.
- You can also layer the pudding with Low-FODMAP fruits for a parfait effect.

Nutritional Value (per serving):

- Calories: 200

- Protein: 5g
- Carbohydrates: 25g
- Fat: 10g
- Fiber: 10g

Scrambled Eggs with Spinach and Feta

Ingredients:

- 2 large eggs
- 1/4 cup lactose-free feta cheese
- 1 cup fresh spinach
- 1 tbsp lactose-free milk or almond milk
- Salt and pepper to taste
- 1 tsp olive oil

Cooking Instructions:

1. In a bowl, whisk together the eggs, milk, salt, and pepper.
2. Heat olive oil in a skillet over medium heat.
3. Add the spinach to the skillet and sauté for 1-2 minutes until wilted.
4. Pour the egg mixture into the skillet and stir gently.
5. As the eggs start to set, add the feta cheese and continue to scramble until fully cooked.
6. Serve immediately.

Cook Tips:

- For a fluffier scramble, use a whisk to incorporate air into the eggs.
- Serve with a slice of Low-FODMAP toast for a complete meal.

Nutritional Value (per serving):

- Calories: 220

- Protein: 16g
- Carbohydrates: 5g
- Fat: 16g
- Fiber: 1g

Overnight Quinoa with Almond Milk

Ingredients:

- 1/2 cup cooked quinoa
- 1 cup almond milk (unsweetened)
- 1 tbsp chia seeds
- 1 tsp vanilla extract
- 1 tbsp maple syrup or stevia (optional)
- 1/4 cup strawberries or blueberries

Cooking Instructions:

1. In a mason jar or bowl, combine the cooked quinoa, almond milk, chia seeds, vanilla extract, and maple syrup.
2. Stir well, cover, and refrigerate overnight.
3. In the morning, stir again and top with fresh strawberries or blueberries.

Cook Tips:

- Make multiple servings in advance for easy grab-and-go breakfasts during the week.
- You can also warm this dish in the microwave if you prefer a hot breakfast.

Nutritional Value (per serving):

- Calories: 300
- Protein: 10g
- Carbohydrates: 45g

- Fat: 8g
- Fiber: 6g

Cinnamon-Spiced Rice Porridge

Ingredients:

- 1/2 cup cooked white rice
- 1 cup lactose-free milk or almond milk
- 1/2 tsp cinnamon
- 1 tbsp maple syrup or brown sugar
- A pinch of salt
- 1/4 cup Low-FODMAP fruit (like strawberries or blueberries)

Cooking Instructions:

1. In a saucepan, combine the cooked rice, milk, cinnamon, maple syrup, and salt.
2. Bring to a simmer over medium heat, stirring occasionally, until the mixture thickens, about 5-7 minutes.
3. Serve warm with Low-FODMAP fruits and an extra sprinkle of cinnamon if desired.

Cook Tips:

- For creamier porridge, use arborio or sushi rice instead of regular white rice.
- Make a big batch and reheat it throughout the week for a quick breakfast option.

Nutritional Value (per serving):

- Calories: 200
- Protein: 6g
- Carbohydrates: 40g
- Fat: 3g
- Fiber: 3g

FODMAP-Friendly Smoothie Bowl

Ingredients:

- 1/2 banana (unripe)
- 1/2 cup lactose-free yogurt
- 1/4 cup almond milk
- 1 tbsp chia seeds
- 1/4 cup blueberries
- 1 tbsp peanut butter (optional)
- Low-FODMAP granola for topping

Cooking Instructions:

1. Blend the banana, yogurt, almond milk, and chia seeds until smooth.
2. Pour into a bowl and top with blueberries, peanut butter, and Low-FODMAP granola.
3. Serve immediately.

Cook Tips:

- Use frozen banana for a creamier, thicker texture.
- You can also top it with coconut flakes for added crunch.

Nutritional Value (per serving):

- Calories: 350
- Protein: 10g
- Carbohydrates: 50g
- Fat: 12g
- Fiber: 8g

Gluten-Free Banana Bread

Ingredients:

- 2 ripe bananas
- 2 eggs
- 1/4 cup coconut oil (melted)
- 1/4 cup maple syrup or honey
- 1 tsp vanilla extract
- 1 1/2 cups gluten-free all-purpose flour
- 1 tsp baking soda
- 1/2 tsp cinnamon
- A pinch of salt

Cooking Instructions:

1. Preheat your oven to 350°F (175°C) and grease a loaf pan with coconut oil.
2. In a large bowl, mash the bananas until smooth. Stir in the eggs, coconut oil, maple syrup, and vanilla extract.
3. In another bowl, whisk together the gluten-free flour, baking soda, cinnamon, and salt.
4. Gradually add the dry ingredients to the wet mixture, stirring until just combined.
5. Pour the batter into the prepared loaf pan and bake for 50-60 minutes or until a toothpick inserted into the center comes out clean.
6. Let the bread cool in the pan for 10 minutes before transferring it to a wire rack to cool completely.

Cook Tips:

- You can fold in Low-FODMAP fruits like blueberries or nuts like walnuts for added texture and flavor.
- To prevent the bread from becoming too dry, store it in an airtight container for up to three days or freeze it for longer storage.

Nutritional Value (per serving):

- Calories: 180
- Protein: 3g
- Carbohydrates: 30g
- Fat: 7g
- Fiber: 2g

Low-FODMAP Granola with Coconut Yogurt

Ingredients:

- 2 cups gluten-free oats
- 1/2 cup chopped almonds
- 1/4 cup shredded coconut (unsweetened)
- 1/4 cup maple syrup or honey
- 2 tbsp coconut oil (melted)
- 1 tsp vanilla extract
- A pinch of cinnamon and salt
- 1 cup coconut yogurt (for serving)

Cooking Instructions:

1. Preheat your oven to 300°F (150°C) and line a baking sheet with parchment paper.
2. In a large bowl, mix together the oats, almonds, shredded coconut, cinnamon, and salt.
3. In a separate bowl, whisk together the maple syrup, coconut oil, and vanilla extract.
4. Pour the wet mixture over the dry ingredients and stir until well combined.
5. Spread the mixture evenly on the prepared baking sheet and bake for 20-25 minutes, stirring halfway through, until golden and crispy.

6. Allow the granola to cool completely before serving with coconut yogurt.

Cook Tips:

- Store leftover granola in an airtight container for up to two weeks.
- You can customize this recipe by adding pumpkin seeds or sunflower seeds for extra crunch.

Nutritional Value (per serving):

- Calories: 320
- Protein: 5g
- Carbohydrates: 45g
- Fat: 15g
- Fiber: 5g

Scrambled Tofu with Bell Peppers

Ingredients:

- 1 block firm tofu (drained and crumbled)
- 1 red bell pepper (diced)
- 1/2 tsp turmeric powder
- 1 tbsp olive oil
- 1 tsp cumin powder
- 1 tbsp nutritional yeast (optional)
- Salt and pepper to taste
- Fresh parsley for garnish

Cooking Instructions:

1. Heat olive oil in a skillet over medium heat.
2. Add the diced bell pepper and sauté for 3-4 minutes until softened.

3. Add the crumbled tofu, turmeric, cumin, salt, and pepper to the skillet, and stir well to combine.

4. Cook for 5-7 minutes, stirring occasionally, until the tofu is heated through and takes on a scrambled egg-like texture.

5. Stir in the nutritional yeast, if using, and garnish with fresh parsley before serving.

Cook Tips:

- Press the tofu before crumbling it to remove excess moisture and improve the texture.
- You can add other Low-FODMAP veggies like spinach or zucchini for variety.

Nutritional Value (per serving):

- Calories: 200
- Protein: 12g
- Carbohydrates: 6g
- Fat: 14g
- Fiber: 3g

Sweet Potato Breakfast Hash

Ingredients:

- 2 medium sweet potatoes (peeled and diced)
- 1 red bell pepper (diced)
- 1 tbsp olive oil
- 1/2 tsp paprika
- 1/2 tsp cumin powder
- Salt and pepper to taste
- 2 eggs (optional for serving)

Cooking Instructions:

1. Preheat your oven to 400°F (200°C) and line a baking sheet with parchment paper.
2. Toss the diced sweet potatoes and bell pepper with olive oil, paprika, cumin, salt, and pepper.
3. Spread the mixture evenly on the baking sheet and roast for 25-30 minutes until the sweet potatoes are tender and golden.
4. If serving with eggs, fry or poach them during the last 5 minutes of roasting time.
5. Serve the roasted sweet potato hash with eggs on top, if desired.

Cook Tips:

- You can add chopped spinach or kale to the hash for extra nutrients.
- Leftovers can be reheated in a skillet the next day for a quick breakfast.

Nutritional Value (per serving):

- Calories: 230
- Protein: 4g
- Carbohydrates: 40g
- Fat: 8g
- Fiber: 6g

Low-FODMAP Pumpkin Muffins

Ingredients:

- 1 cup gluten-free flour
- 1/2 cup pumpkin puree (canned or homemade)
- 2 eggs
- 1/4 cup maple syrup
- 1/4 cup coconut oil (melted)

- 1 tsp vanilla extract
- 1 tsp cinnamon
- 1/2 tsp baking soda
- A pinch of salt

Cooking Instructions:

1. Preheat your oven to 350°F (175°C) and line a muffin tin with paper liners.
2. In a large bowl, whisk together the pumpkin puree, eggs, maple syrup, coconut oil, and vanilla extract.
3. In another bowl, combine the gluten-free flour, cinnamon, baking soda, and salt.
4. Add the dry ingredients to the wet mixture and stir until just combined.
5. Divide the batter evenly among the muffin cups and bake for 20-25 minutes, or until a toothpick inserted in the center comes out clean.
6. Let the muffins cool in the pan for 5 minutes before transferring them to a wire rack to cool completely.

Cook Tips:

- You can add Low-FODMAP chocolate chips or chopped walnuts to the batter for extra flavor.
- These muffins freeze well, making them perfect for meal prep.

Nutritional Value (per muffin):

- Calories: 150
- Protein: 3g
- Carbohydrates: 20g
- Fat: 7g
- Fiber: 2g

Warm Buckwheat Porridge with Chia Seeds

Ingredients:

- 1/2 cup buckwheat groats
- 1 1/2 cups lactose-free milk or almond milk
- 1 tbsp chia seeds
- 1 tsp vanilla extract
- 1 tbsp maple syrup (optional)
- 1/4 cup Low-FODMAP fruits like strawberries or blueberries

Cooking Instructions:

1. Rinse the buckwheat groats under cold water, then add them to a saucepan with the milk.
2. Bring the mixture to a simmer over medium heat and cook for 10-12 minutes, stirring occasionally, until the buckwheat is tender and the milk is absorbed.
3. Stir in the chia seeds, vanilla extract, and maple syrup, if using.
4. Serve the porridge warm with Low-FODMAP fruits on top.

Cook Tips:

- Soak the buckwheat groats overnight to reduce the cooking time in the morning.
- You can add a sprinkle of cinnamon or nutmeg for extra flavor.

Nutritional Value (per serving):

- Calories: 250
- Protein: 8g
- Carbohydrates: 45g
- Fat: 5g
- Fiber: 8g

Chapter 2: Nourishing Lunches for Digestive Ease

Quinoa and Kale Salad with Lemon Dressing

Ingredients:

- 1 cup cooked quinoa
- 2 cups kale, chopped
- 1/4 cup cherry tomatoes, halved
- 1/4 cup cucumber, diced
- 1/4 cup shredded carrots
- 2 tbsp olive oil
- 2 tbsp lemon juice
- 1 tsp Dijon mustard
- Salt and pepper to taste

Cooking Instructions:

1. In a large bowl, combine the cooked quinoa, kale, cherry tomatoes, cucumber, and shredded carrots.
2. In a small bowl, whisk together the olive oil, lemon juice, Dijon mustard, salt, and pepper.
3. Pour the dressing over the salad and toss to combine. Let the salad sit for 10 minutes before serving to allow the kale to soften.

Cook Tips:

- Massage the kale with a little olive oil before adding it to the salad to make it more tender.
- Add a sprinkle of Low-FODMAP seeds like sunflower or pumpkin for extra crunch.

Nutritional Value (per serving):

- Calories: 320
- Protein: 8g
- Carbohydrates: 40g
- Fat: 16g
- Fiber: 6g

Grilled Chicken Caesar Salad (Low-FODMAP Dressing)

Ingredients:

- 2 boneless, skinless chicken breasts
- 4 cups romaine lettuce, chopped
- 1/4 cup grated Parmesan cheese
- 1/4 cup gluten-free croutons (optional)

Dressing Ingredients:

- 1/4 cup mayonnaise (Low-FODMAP)
- 1 tbsp Dijon mustard
- 1 tbsp lemon juice
- 1 tsp anchovy paste (optional)
- 1/2 tsp garlic-infused oil
- Salt and pepper to taste

Cooking Instructions:

1. Season the chicken breasts with salt and pepper, and grill them over medium heat for 6-7 minutes on each side until fully cooked. Let the chicken rest for 5 minutes, then slice.
2. In a small bowl, whisk together all the dressing ingredients until smooth.

3. In a large bowl, toss the romaine lettuce with the dressing, then top with grilled chicken, Parmesan cheese, and croutons.

4. Serve immediately.

Cook Tips:

- For a more authentic Caesar dressing, use anchovy paste, but it can be omitted for a milder flavor.
- If grilling isn't an option, pan-fry or bake the chicken for similar results.

Nutritional Value (per serving):

- Calories: 450
- Protein: 36g
- Carbohydrates: 12g
- Fat: 26g
- Fiber: 4g

Gluten-Free Turkey Wraps with Cucumber and Carrots

Ingredients:

- 4 gluten-free tortillas
- 8 slices deli turkey (Low-FODMAP certified)
- 1/2 cucumber, julienned
- 1/2 carrot, shredded
- 1/4 cup lactose-free cream cheese
- 1 tbsp Dijon mustard
- Salt and pepper to taste

Cooking Instructions:

1. Spread a thin layer of lactose-free cream cheese over each tortilla.
2. Layer the turkey slices, cucumber, and shredded carrot on each tortilla.

3. Drizzle with a little Dijon mustard, and season with salt and pepper.

4. Roll each tortilla tightly into a wrap and slice in half to serve.

Cook Tips:

- You can add spinach or lettuce for more crunch and nutrition.
- Wraps can be prepared ahead and stored in the fridge for up to 24 hours.

Nutritional Value (per wrap):

- Calories: 280
- Protein: 18g
- Carbohydrates: 32g
- Fat: 9g
- Fiber: 3g

Low-FODMAP Mediterranean Chickpea Salad

Ingredients:

- 1 can chickpeas (drained and rinsed)
- 1/2 cup cherry tomatoes, halved
- 1/4 cup cucumber, diced
- 1/4 cup feta cheese (lactose-free)
- 1/4 cup Kalamata olives, pitted
- 2 tbsp olive oil
- 1 tbsp red wine vinegar
- 1 tsp oregano
- Salt and pepper to taste

Cooking Instructions:

1. In a large bowl, combine the chickpeas, cherry tomatoes, cucumber, feta cheese, and Kalamata olives.

2. In a small bowl, whisk together the olive oil, red wine vinegar, oregano, salt, and pepper.

3. Pour the dressing over the salad and toss to combine. Serve chilled or at room temperature.

Cook Tips:

- Let the salad sit for at least 10 minutes to allow the flavors to meld.
- This salad makes an excellent meal prep option, as it stores well in the fridge for up to three days.

Nutritional Value (per serving):

- Calories: 320
- Protein: 10g
- Carbohydrates: 36g
- Fat: 16g
- Fiber: 8g

Zucchini Noodles with Pesto and Grilled Shrimp

Ingredients:

- 4 medium zucchini (spiralized into noodles)
- 12 large shrimp (peeled and deveined)
- 1/4 cup Low-FODMAP pesto (store-bought or homemade)
- 2 tbsp olive oil
- Salt and pepper to taste

Cooking Instructions:

1. Preheat a grill or grill pan over medium heat. Toss the shrimp with 1 tbsp olive oil, salt, and pepper. Grill for 2-3 minutes on each side until cooked through.

2. In a large skillet, heat the remaining 1 tbsp olive oil over medium heat. Add the zucchini noodles and sauté for 2-3 minutes until just tender.

3. Toss the zucchini noodles with the pesto, and top with the grilled shrimp. Serve immediately.

Cook Tips:

- Be careful not to overcook the zucchini noodles, as they can become mushy.
- If you don't have a grill, pan-fry the shrimp until they are opaque and fully cooked.

Nutritional Value (per serving):

- Calories: 290
- Protein: 24g
- Carbohydrates: 12g
- Fat: 18g
- Fiber: 4g

Tuna and Avocado Salad with Lemon Vinaigrette

Ingredients:

- 1 can tuna (in water, drained)
- 1 ripe avocado (cubed)
- 1/4 cup cucumber, diced
- 1 tbsp lemon juice
- 2 tbsp olive oil
- 1 tsp Dijon mustard
- Salt and pepper to taste

Cooking Instructions:

1. In a medium bowl, combine the drained tuna, cubed avocado, and cucumber.

2. In a small bowl, whisk together the lemon juice, olive oil, Dijon mustard, salt, and pepper.

3. Pour the dressing over the salad and gently toss to combine. Serve immediately.

Cook Tips:

- Serve this salad in a lettuce wrap or with gluten-free crackers for added texture.
- For extra flavor, sprinkle with chopped fresh herbs like parsley or dill.

Nutritional Value (per serving):

- Calories: 320
- Protein: 20g
- Carbohydrates: 10g
- Fat: 24g
- Fiber: 6g

Low-FODMAP Chicken and Rice Stir-Fry

Ingredients:

- 2 boneless, skinless chicken breasts (sliced into thin strips)
- 2 cups cooked white rice
- 1 red bell pepper, sliced
- 1 zucchini, sliced
- 1 tbsp garlic-infused oil
- 2 tbsp tamari (gluten-free soy sauce)
- 1 tbsp sesame oil
- Salt and pepper to taste

Cooking Instructions:

1. Heat the garlic-infused oil in a large skillet over medium heat. Add the chicken strips and cook until golden brown, about 5-7 minutes.

2. Add the bell pepper and zucchini to the skillet and cook for another 3-4 minutes until tender.

3. Stir in the tamari, sesame oil, and cooked rice, tossing everything together. Cook for 2-3 minutes until heated through.

4. Season with salt and pepper to taste and serve immediately.

Cook Tips:

- Add Low-FODMAP-friendly herbs like cilantro or parsley for extra flavor.
- This stir-fry is highly versatile, so you can swap out the vegetables based on what you have on hand.

Nutritional Value (per serving):

- Calories: 380
- Protein: 28g
- Carbohydrates: 45g
- Fat: 12g
- Fiber: 4g

Lentil and Sweet Potato Soup

Ingredients:

- 1 cup red lentils, rinsed
- 1 large sweet potato, peeled and diced
- 1 carrot, chopped
- 1 tbsp garlic-infused olive oil
- 4 cups low-sodium vegetable broth
- 1 tsp ground cumin
- 1/2 tsp turmeric
- Salt and pepper to taste

Cooking Instructions:

1. In a large pot, heat the garlic-infused olive oil over medium heat. Add the diced sweet potato and carrot, and sauté for 5 minutes.
2. Add the lentils, cumin, turmeric, and vegetable broth. Stir well to combine.
3. Bring the soup to a boil, then reduce the heat to low and simmer for 20-25 minutes, until the lentils and sweet potato are tender.
4. Season with salt and pepper to taste. Serve warm.

Cook Tips:

- For a creamier texture, blend half the soup with an immersion blender and mix it back into the pot.
- This soup can be stored in the fridge for up to four days or frozen for later use.

Nutritional Value (per serving):

- Calories: 280
- Protein: 13g
- Carbohydrates: 52g
- Fat: 5g
- Fiber: 14g

Roasted Vegetable Quinoa Bowl

Ingredients:

- 1 cup cooked quinoa
- 1 zucchini, diced
- 1 red bell pepper, diced
- 1 carrot, diced
- 1 tbsp olive oil
- 1/2 tsp paprika

- Salt and pepper to taste

Cooking Instructions:

1. Preheat your oven to 400°F (200°C) and line a baking sheet with parchment paper.
2. Toss the diced zucchini, bell pepper, and carrot with olive oil, paprika, salt, and pepper. Spread the vegetables evenly on the baking sheet.
3. Roast the vegetables for 20-25 minutes, stirring halfway through, until they are tender and slightly caramelized.
4. In a bowl, combine the roasted vegetables with the cooked quinoa. Serve warm.

Cook Tips:

- You can switch up the vegetables based on what's in season or your personal preference.
- Add a drizzle of tahini or a sprinkle of feta cheese for extra flavor.

Nutritional Value (per serving):

- Calories: 300
- Protein: 8g
- Carbohydrates: 45g
- Fat: 10g
- Fiber: 7g

Low-FODMAP Spinach and Feta Wrap

Ingredients:

- 4 gluten-free wraps
- 2 cups fresh spinach
- 1/4 cup lactose-free feta cheese
- 2 tbsp garlic-infused olive oil

- Salt and pepper to taste

Cooking Instructions:

1. In a skillet, heat the garlic-infused olive oil over medium heat. Add the spinach and sauté for 2-3 minutes until wilted. Season with salt and pepper.
2. Divide the sautéed spinach and feta cheese evenly among the gluten-free wraps.
3. Roll up the wraps tightly and serve warm or at room temperature.

Cook Tips:

- For a warm, crispy wrap, heat the assembled wrap in a pan for 1-2 minutes on each side.
- You can add some roasted red peppers for extra flavor and color.

Nutritional Value (per wrap):

- Calories: 250
- Protein: 10g
- Carbohydrates: 30g
- Fat: 12g
- Fiber: 4g

Baked Salmon with Herbed Quinoa

Ingredients:

- 2 salmon fillets
- 1 cup cooked quinoa
- 1 tbsp olive oil
- 1 tbsp lemon juice
- 1 tsp dried oregano
- 1 tsp dried basil
- Salt and pepper to taste

Cooking Instructions:

1. Preheat your oven to 375°F (190°C) and line a baking sheet with parchment paper.
2. Season the salmon fillets with olive oil, lemon juice, oregano, basil, salt, and pepper. Place them on the prepared baking sheet.
3. Bake the salmon for 15-20 minutes, or until the fish flakes easily with a fork.
4. Serve the salmon over a bed of cooked quinoa and garnish with fresh herbs.

Cook Tips:

- Pair this dish with a side of steamed vegetables or a fresh green salad for a complete meal.
- Add a squeeze of fresh lemon juice just before serving for a burst of flavor.

Nutritional Value (per serving):

- Calories: 380
- Protein: 32g
- Carbohydrates: 25g
- Fat: 18g
- Fiber: 4g

Roasted Carrot Soup with Ginger

Ingredients:

- 4 large carrots, peeled and chopped
- 1 tbsp fresh ginger, grated
- 1 tbsp garlic-infused olive oil
- 4 cups low-sodium vegetable broth
- Salt and pepper to taste

Cooking Instructions:

1. Preheat your oven to 400°F (200°C) and line a baking sheet with parchment paper.
2. Toss the chopped carrots with garlic-infused olive oil, salt, and pepper, then spread them evenly on the baking sheet.
3. Roast the carrots for 25-30 minutes, until tender and slightly caramelized.
4. In a large pot, combine the roasted carrots, ginger, and vegetable broth. Bring to a simmer and cook for 10 minutes.
5. Use an immersion blender to puree the soup until smooth. Season with additional salt and pepper to taste.

Cook Tips:

- Add a dollop of lactose-free yogurt or coconut cream on top for a creamy finish.
- This soup freezes well, making it great for meal prep.

Nutritional Value (per serving):

- Calories: 180
- Protein: 3g
- Carbohydrates: 28g
- Fat: 8g
- Fiber: 6g

Turkey and Spinach Frittata

Ingredients:

- 6 large eggs
- 1/2 cup cooked ground turkey
- 1 cup fresh spinach, chopped
- 1/4 cup lactose-free cheddar cheese, shredded

- 1 tbsp olive oil
- Salt and pepper to taste

Cooking Instructions:

1. Preheat your oven to 350°F (175°C).
2. In a bowl, whisk together the eggs, salt, and pepper.
3. In a skillet, heat the olive oil over medium heat. Add the ground turkey and spinach, cooking until the spinach wilts and the turkey is heated through.
4. Pour the egg mixture over the turkey and spinach, then sprinkle the cheese on top.
5. Transfer the skillet to the oven and bake for 15-20 minutes, or until the frittata is set and slightly golden.
6. Slice and serve warm.

Cook Tips:

- Use a cast iron skillet for even cooking and an easy transition from stovetop to oven.
- Leftover frittata makes a great breakfast or snack the next day.

Nutritional Value (per serving):

- Calories: 250
- Protein: 20g
- Carbohydrates: 2g
- Fat: 18g
- Fiber: 1g

Soba Noodle Salad with Sesame Dressing

Ingredients:

- 6 oz gluten-free soba noodles

- 1/2 cucumber, thinly sliced
- 1/2 red bell pepper, thinly sliced
- 2 tbsp sesame oil
- 1 tbsp tamari (gluten-free soy sauce)
- 1 tbsp rice vinegar
- 1 tsp maple syrup
- 1 tsp sesame seeds
- Salt and pepper to taste

Cooking Instructions:

1. Cook the soba noodles according to package instructions, then rinse under cold water and drain.
2. In a small bowl, whisk together the sesame oil, tamari, rice vinegar, maple syrup, sesame seeds, salt, and pepper.
3. Toss the cooked soba noodles with the cucumber, bell pepper, and dressing until well combined.
4. Serve chilled or at room temperature.

Cook Tips:

- Add grilled shrimp or tofu for extra protein.
- Garnish with fresh cilantro or green onions for added freshness.

Nutritional Value (per serving):

- Calories: 350
- Protein: 10g
- Carbohydrates: 50g
- Fat: 12g
- Fiber: 5g

Grilled Vegetable Panini (Low-FODMAP Bread)

Ingredients:

- 4 slices Low-FODMAP bread
- 1/2 zucchini, sliced
- 1/4 red bell pepper, sliced
- 1 tbsp olive oil
- 1/4 cup lactose-free mozzarella cheese, shredded
- 1 tbsp pesto (Low-FODMAP)
- Salt and pepper to taste

Cooking Instructions:

1. Heat a grill pan over medium heat and lightly brush the zucchini and bell pepper slices with olive oil. Grill for 3-4 minutes on each side until tender.
2. Spread pesto on two slices of Low-FODMAP bread, then layer the grilled vegetables and mozzarella cheese on top. Season with salt and pepper.
3. Top with the remaining bread slices and press the sandwiches in a panini press or grill pan for 2-3 minutes on each side until golden and the cheese is melted.
4. Serve warm.

Cook Tips:

- For extra flavor, you can add fresh basil leaves or a drizzle of balsamic glaze.
- If you don't have a panini press, you can use a regular skillet with another heavy pan to press the sandwich.

Nutritional Value (per serving):

- Calories: 320
- Protein: 12g
- Carbohydrates: 40g
- Fat: 12g
- Fiber: 4g

Chapter 3: Satisfying Dinners for Symptom-Free Evenings

Lemon Herb Chicken with Roasted Potatoes

Ingredients:

- 2 boneless, skinless chicken breasts
- 4 medium potatoes, diced
- 2 tbsp olive oil
- 2 tbsp lemon juice
- 1 tbsp fresh parsley, chopped
- 1 tsp dried thyme
- Salt and pepper to taste

Cooking Instructions:

1. Preheat your oven to 400°F (200°C).
2. In a bowl, toss the diced potatoes with 1 tbsp olive oil, salt, and pepper. Spread them on a baking sheet and roast for 20-25 minutes, flipping halfway.
3. While the potatoes are roasting, heat the remaining olive oil in a skillet over medium heat. Season the chicken breasts with salt, pepper, thyme, and lemon juice.
4. Cook the chicken for 6-7 minutes on each side until golden and cooked through.
5. Once done, remove the chicken and let it rest for 5 minutes before slicing. Sprinkle with parsley and serve with roasted potatoes.

Cook Tips:

- You can also add roasted carrots or zucchini for extra veggies.
- Marinate the chicken in the lemon and herb mixture for a few hours to enhance the flavors.

Nutritional Value (per serving):

- Calories: 400
- Protein: 35g
- Carbohydrates: 40g
- Fat: 14g
- Fiber: 5g

Baked Cod with Asparagus and Lemon Sauce

Ingredients:

- 2 cod fillets
- 1 bunch asparagus, trimmed
- 2 tbsp olive oil
- 2 tbsp lemon juice
- 1 tsp Dijon mustard
- 1 tsp garlic-infused oil
- Salt and pepper to taste

Cooking Instructions:

1. Preheat your oven to 375°F (190°C).
2. In a small bowl, whisk together the olive oil, lemon juice, Dijon mustard, and garlic-infused oil.
3. Place the cod fillets and asparagus on a baking sheet lined with parchment paper. Drizzle the lemon sauce over the fish and vegetables.
4. Bake for 15-20 minutes, until the fish flakes easily with a fork and the asparagus is tender.
5. Serve immediately, garnished with extra lemon slices.

Cook Tips:

- Add fresh herbs like parsley or dill for extra flavor.
- This dish pairs well with quinoa or rice for a balanced meal.

Nutritional Value (per serving):

- Calories: 280
- Protein: 28g
- Carbohydrates: 6g
- Fat: 14g
- Fiber: 4g

Low-FODMAP Beef Stir-Fry with Broccoli

Ingredients:

- 8 oz beef sirloin, thinly sliced
- 2 cups broccoli florets
- 2 tbsp tamari (gluten-free soy sauce)
- 1 tbsp sesame oil
- 1 tsp garlic-infused oil
- 1 tsp fresh ginger, grated
- Salt and pepper to taste

Cooking Instructions:

1. Heat the sesame oil in a large skillet over medium heat. Add the sliced beef and cook for 4-5 minutes until browned.
2. Add the broccoli and cook for another 3-4 minutes until tender-crisp.
3. Stir in the tamari, garlic-infused oil, and grated ginger. Cook for an additional 2 minutes until everything is coated and heated through.
4. Season with salt and pepper to taste and serve immediately.

Cook Tips:

- Serve with steamed rice or gluten-free noodles for a complete meal.
- Add red bell pepper or carrots for more color and nutrients.

Nutritional Value (per serving):

- Calories: 350
- Protein: 30g
- Carbohydrates: 10g
- Fat: 20g
- Fiber: 4g

Zucchini Lasagna with Ricotta and Spinach

Ingredients:

- 2 large zucchinis, sliced thin lengthwise
- 1 cup ricotta cheese (lactose-free)
- 1/2 cup spinach, chopped
- 1 egg
- 1 cup marinara sauce (Low-FODMAP)
- 1/2 cup mozzarella cheese (lactose-free)
- Salt and pepper to taste

Cooking Instructions:

1. Preheat your oven to 375°F (190°C).
2. In a bowl, mix the ricotta cheese, spinach, egg, salt, and pepper.
3. In a baking dish, layer the zucchini slices, ricotta mixture, and marinara sauce. Repeat until all ingredients are used, ending with marinara sauce on top.
4. Sprinkle the mozzarella cheese on top and bake for 25-30 minutes until the cheese is bubbly and golden.

5. Let it cool for 5 minutes before serving.

Cook Tips:

- Use a mandoline slicer to get even zucchini slices.
- This lasagna can be stored in the fridge for up to 3 days or frozen for future meals.

Nutritional Value (per serving):

- Calories: 320
- Protein: 20g
- Carbohydrates: 12g
- Fat: 22g
- Fiber: 4g

Grilled Pork Chops with Sweet Potato Mash

Ingredients:

- 2 bone-in pork chops
- 2 medium sweet potatoes, peeled and diced
- 1 tbsp olive oil
- 1 tbsp fresh rosemary, chopped
- 1 tbsp butter (lactose-free)
- Salt and pepper to taste

Cooking Instructions:

1. Boil the sweet potatoes in salted water for 10-12 minutes, until tender. Drain and mash with butter, salt, and pepper.
2. Meanwhile, heat the olive oil in a skillet over medium heat. Season the pork chops with rosemary, salt, and pepper.

3. Grill the pork chops for 4-5 minutes on each side until fully cooked and juices run clear.

4. Serve the pork chops with sweet potato mash on the side.

Cook Tips:

- Let the pork chops rest for 5 minutes after grilling to retain moisture.
- Add a side of steamed green beans or a simple salad for a balanced meal.

Nutritional Value (per serving):

- Calories: 450
- Protein: 35g
- Carbohydrates: 40g
- Fat: 18g
- Fiber: 6g

Baked Eggplant Parmesan (Gluten-Free)

Ingredients:

- 1 large eggplant, sliced into rounds
- 1 cup gluten-free breadcrumbs
- 1/2 cup grated Parmesan cheese
- 1 cup marinara sauce (Low-FODMAP)
- 1 cup mozzarella cheese (lactose-free)
- 1 egg, beaten
- Salt and pepper to taste

Cooking Instructions:

1. Preheat your oven to 375°F (190°C) and line a baking sheet with parchment paper.

2. Dip each eggplant slice into the beaten egg, then coat with a mixture of gluten-free breadcrumbs, Parmesan cheese, salt, and pepper.

3. Place the breaded eggplant slices on the baking sheet and bake for 20-25 minutes, flipping halfway, until golden and crispy.

4. In a baking dish, layer the baked eggplant with marinara sauce and mozzarella cheese. Bake for an additional 15-20 minutes until the cheese is melted and bubbly.

5. Serve warm.

Cook Tips:

- For extra crispiness, broil the eggplant for the last 2-3 minutes of baking.
- This dish pairs well with gluten-free pasta or a side salad.

Nutritional Value (per serving):

- Calories: 350
- Protein: 20g
- Carbohydrates: 40g
- Fat: 15g
- Fiber: 7g

Lemon and Herb Grilled Salmon with Rice

Ingredients:

- 2 salmon fillets
- 1 cup cooked white rice
- 2 tbsp olive oil
- 1 tbsp lemon juice
- 1 tsp fresh dill, chopped
- Salt and pepper to taste

Cooking Instructions:

1. Preheat your grill to medium heat. Brush the salmon fillets with olive oil, lemon juice, dill, salt, and pepper.
2. Grill the salmon for 5-6 minutes on each side until it flakes easily with a fork.
3. Serve the grilled salmon over a bed of cooked white rice with extra lemon slices on the side.

Cook Tips:

- If grilling isn't an option, bake the salmon in the oven at 375°F (190°C) for 15-20 minutes.
- Add steamed vegetables like broccoli or asparagus for a well-rounded meal.

Nutritional Value (per serving):

- Calories: 400
- Protein: 35g
- Carbohydrates: 30g
- Fat: 18g
- Fiber: 2g

Turkey Meatballs with Zucchini Noodles

Ingredients:

- 1 lb ground turkey
- 1/4 cup gluten-free breadcrumbs
- 1 egg
- 1 tbsp fresh parsley, chopped
- 1 tsp oregano
- 4 medium zucchini (spiralized into noodles)
- 2 tbsp olive oil

- 1 cup marinara sauce (Low-FODMAP)
- Salt and pepper to taste

Cooking Instructions:

1. Preheat your oven to 375°F (190°C). In a bowl, combine the ground turkey, breadcrumbs, egg, parsley, oregano, salt, and pepper. Mix well and form into meatballs.
2. Place the meatballs on a baking sheet and bake for 20-25 minutes until fully cooked.
3. Meanwhile, heat olive oil in a skillet and sauté the zucchini noodles for 2-3 minutes until tender.
4. Serve the meatballs over the zucchini noodles, topped with marinara sauce.

Cook Tips:

- Make a large batch of meatballs and freeze them for quick meals later.
- Add grated Parmesan cheese on top for extra flavor.

Nutritional Value (per serving):

- Calories: 350
- Protein: 28g
- Carbohydrates: 15g
- Fat: 18g
- Fiber: 4g

Garlic-Infused Shrimp and Grits (FODMAP-Free)

Ingredients:

- 12 large shrimp (peeled and deveined)
- 1/2 cup grits (polenta)
- 1 cup lactose-free milk or water
- 1 tbsp garlic-infused oil

- 1 tbsp butter (lactose-free)
- 1/2 tsp paprika
- 1 tsp lemon juice
- Salt and pepper to taste

Cooking Instructions:

1. Cook the grits according to package instructions, using lactose-free milk or water. Once cooked, stir in the butter, salt, and pepper, and set aside.
2. In a skillet, heat the garlic-infused oil over medium heat. Add the shrimp, paprika, lemon juice, salt, and pepper. Cook for 2-3 minutes on each side until the shrimp are opaque and cooked through.
3. Serve the shrimp over the warm grits.

Cook Tips:

- For extra flavor, add a pinch of cayenne pepper to the shrimp for some heat.
- Pair with a side of sautéed spinach or collard greens for a well-rounded meal.

Nutritional Value (per serving):

- Calories: 320
- Protein: 25g
- Carbohydrates: 30g
- Fat: 12g
- Fiber: 3g

Slow-Cooked Chicken Tacos (Low-FODMAP Wrap)

Ingredients:

- 2 boneless, skinless chicken breasts
- 1 tsp paprika
- 1 tsp cumin

- 1 tsp chili powder
- 1/2 tsp salt
- 1/2 tsp pepper
- 1/2 cup Low-FODMAP salsa
- 8 Low-FODMAP tortillas
- 1/4 cup lactose-free sour cream
- Fresh cilantro for garnish

Cooking Instructions:

1. In a slow cooker, place the chicken breasts and sprinkle with paprika, cumin, chili powder, salt, and pepper. Pour the Low-FODMAP salsa on top.
2. Cook on low for 6 hours or on high for 3 hours until the chicken is tender and easy to shred.
3. Shred the chicken with two forks, then stir it back into the sauce.
4. Serve the shredded chicken in Low-FODMAP tortillas with lactose-free sour cream and fresh cilantro.

Cook Tips:

- Make extra chicken and use the leftovers for salads or burrito bowls.
- Top the tacos with Low-FODMAP veggies like shredded lettuce, cucumber, or chopped tomatoes.

Nutritional Value (per taco):

- Calories: 250
- Protein: 22g
- Carbohydrates: 20g
- Fat: 8g
- Fiber: 3g

Grilled Vegetable Skewers with Quinoa

Ingredients:

- 1 zucchini, sliced into rounds
- 1 red bell pepper, cut into chunks
- 1 yellow bell pepper, cut into chunks
- 1 tbsp olive oil
- 1 tbsp lemon juice
- 1 tsp dried oregano
- Salt and pepper to taste
- 1 cup cooked quinoa

Cooking Instructions:

1. Preheat your grill or grill pan to medium heat.
2. Thread the zucchini, red bell pepper, and yellow bell pepper onto skewers. Brush with olive oil, lemon juice, oregano, salt, and pepper.
3. Grill the skewers for 5-7 minutes on each side until the vegetables are tender and lightly charred.
4. Serve the grilled vegetables over cooked quinoa.

Cook Tips:

- For extra flavor, marinate the vegetables in the oil and lemon juice mixture for 30 minutes before grilling.
- Add fresh herbs like parsley or mint to the quinoa for a fresh twist.

Nutritional Value (per serving):

- Calories: 290
- Protein: 8g
- Carbohydrates: 40g
- Fat: 10g
- Fiber: 6g

Beef and Sweet Potato Shepherd's Pie

Ingredients:

- 1 lb ground beef (lean)
- 1 large sweet potato, peeled and diced
- 1/2 cup carrots, diced
- 1/2 cup green beans, chopped
- 1 tbsp garlic-infused oil
- 1 tbsp tomato paste
- 1/2 cup beef broth (Low-FODMAP)
- Salt and pepper to taste

Cooking Instructions:

1. Preheat your oven to 375°F (190°C).
2. Boil the sweet potatoes in salted water for 10-12 minutes, until tender. Drain, mash with a little butter, salt, and pepper, and set aside.
3. In a skillet, heat the garlic-infused oil and cook the ground beef until browned. Add the carrots and green beans and cook for another 5 minutes.
4. Stir in the tomato paste and beef broth, season with salt and pepper, and simmer for 10 minutes.
5. Transfer the beef mixture to a baking dish, spread the mashed sweet potatoes on top, and bake for 20-25 minutes until golden.

Cook Tips:

- Add a sprinkle of lactose-free cheese on top of the mashed sweet potatoes for extra richness.
- This dish can be prepared ahead of time and baked just before serving.

Nutritional Value (per serving):

- Calories: 380
- Protein: 28g
- Carbohydrates: 30g
- Fat: 18g
- Fiber: 5g

Spinach and Ricotta-Stuffed Bell Peppers

Ingredients:

- 4 large bell peppers, tops cut off and seeds removed
- 1 cup fresh spinach, chopped
- 1/2 cup ricotta cheese (lactose-free)
- 1/4 cup grated Parmesan cheese
- 1 egg
- Salt and pepper to taste

Cooking Instructions:

1. Preheat your oven to 375°F (190°C).
2. In a bowl, mix together the spinach, ricotta, Parmesan, egg, salt, and pepper.
3. Stuff each bell pepper with the spinach and ricotta mixture, then place them in a baking dish.
4. Cover with foil and bake for 25-30 minutes until the peppers are tender and the filling is set.
5. Serve warm, garnished with fresh herbs if desired.

Cook Tips:

- For a complete meal, serve the stuffed peppers with a side of quinoa or brown rice.

- You can also add some cooked ground turkey or chicken to the filling for extra protein.

Nutritional Value (per serving):

- Calories: 220
- Protein: 12g
- Carbohydrates: 15g
- Fat: 12g
- Fiber: 4g

Gluten-Free Chicken Alfredo with Zoodles

Ingredients:

- 2 boneless, skinless chicken breasts
- 4 medium zucchini, spiralized into noodles
- 1/2 cup lactose-free heavy cream
- 1/4 cup grated Parmesan cheese
- 1 tbsp garlic-infused oil
- 1 tbsp butter (lactose-free)
- Salt and pepper to taste

Cooking Instructions:

1. Season the chicken breasts with salt and pepper. Heat the garlic-infused oil in a skillet and cook the chicken for 6-7 minutes on each side until fully cooked. Remove and slice.
2. In the same skillet, melt the butter and add the lactose-free heavy cream. Simmer for 2-3 minutes until slightly thickened. Stir in the Parmesan cheese and season with salt and pepper.
3. Add the spiralized zucchini noodles to the skillet and toss to coat in the sauce. Cook for 2-3 minutes until the zoodles are tender.

4. Serve the zoodles topped with sliced chicken.

Cook Tips:

- For a more traditional Alfredo, you can use gluten-free pasta instead of zoodles.
- Garnish with fresh parsley or basil for added flavor and color.

Nutritional Value (per serving):

- Calories: 360
- Protein: 30g
- Carbohydrates: 10g
- Fat: 22g
- Fiber: 3g

Roasted Turkey Breast with Cranberry Sauce

Ingredients:

- 1 small turkey breast (about 2-3 lbs)
- 2 tbsp olive oil
- 1 tbsp fresh rosemary, chopped
- 1 tsp dried thyme
- Salt and pepper to taste

For the Cranberry Sauce:

- 1/2 cup fresh cranberries
- 1/4 cup orange juice
- 2 tbsp maple syrup
- 1/4 cup water

Cooking Instructions:

1. Preheat your oven to 350°F (175°C).
2. Rub the turkey breast with olive oil, rosemary, thyme, salt, and pepper. Place the turkey on a roasting pan and roast for 1-1.5 hours, until the internal temperature reaches 165°F (74°C).
3. While the turkey is roasting, prepare the cranberry sauce by combining the cranberries, orange juice, maple syrup, and water in a saucepan. Simmer over medium heat until the cranberries burst and the sauce thickens, about 10 minutes.
4. Let the turkey rest for 10 minutes before slicing. Serve with the cranberry sauce.

Cook Tips:

- For a crispy skin, broil the turkey for the last 5 minutes of roasting.
- Leftover turkey can be used in sandwiches or salads.

Nutritional Value (per serving):

- Calories: 400
- Protein: 45g
- Carbohydrates: 10g
- Fat: 20g
- Fiber: 1g

Chapter 4: Snacks and Small Bites to Keep You Going

Baked Sweet Potato Chips with Sea Salt

Ingredients:

- 2 medium sweet potatoes, thinly sliced
- 1 tbsp olive oil
- 1/2 tsp sea salt

Cooking Instructions:

1. Preheat your oven to 375°F (190°C) and line a baking sheet with parchment paper.
2. Toss the sweet potato slices with olive oil and sea salt until evenly coated.
3. Spread the slices in a single layer on the baking sheet.
4. Bake for 15-20 minutes, flipping halfway through, until the chips are crispy and lightly browned.
5. Let cool before serving.

Cook Tips:

- Use a mandoline slicer for even, thin slices.
- For extra flavor, sprinkle with paprika or garlic powder before baking.

Nutritional Value (per serving):

- Calories: 150
- Protein: 2g
- Carbohydrates: 30g
- Fat: 5g
- Fiber: 4g

Roasted Almonds with Paprika

Ingredients:

- 1 cup raw almonds
- 1 tbsp olive oil
- 1 tsp smoked paprika
- 1/2 tsp sea salt

Cooking Instructions:

1. Preheat your oven to 350°F (175°C) and line a baking sheet with parchment paper.
2. Toss the almonds with olive oil, smoked paprika, and sea salt until evenly coated.
3. Spread the almonds on the baking sheet in a single layer.
4. Roast for 10-12 minutes, stirring once, until fragrant and lightly browned.
5. Let cool before serving.

Cook Tips:

- Store the almonds in an airtight container to keep them fresh for up to two weeks.
- Add a pinch of cayenne pepper for a spicy kick.

Nutritional Value (per serving):

- Calories: 200
- Protein: 6g
- Carbohydrates: 6g
- Fat: 18g
- Fiber: 4g

Low-FODMAP Hummus with Carrot Sticks

Ingredients:

- 1 can chickpeas (drained and rinsed)
- 1/4 cup tahini
- 1 tbsp lemon juice
- 2 tbsp garlic-infused olive oil
- 1/4 cup water
- 1/2 tsp cumin
- Salt and pepper to taste
- 4 medium carrots, cut into sticks

Cooking Instructions:

1. In a food processor, blend the chickpeas, tahini, lemon juice, garlic-infused olive oil, water, cumin, salt, and pepper until smooth.
2. Adjust the consistency by adding more water if needed.
3. Serve with carrot sticks on the side.

Cook Tips:

- Store leftover hummus in an airtight container in the fridge for up to 5 days.
- You can also serve the hummus with cucumber slices or gluten-free crackers.

Nutritional Value (per serving):

- Calories: 250
- Protein: 8g
- Carbohydrates: 25g
- Fat: 12g
- Fiber: 8g

Rice Cakes with Peanut Butter and Banana Slices

Ingredients:

- 4 rice cakes (Low-FODMAP)
- 4 tbsp natural peanut butter
- 1 small banana, sliced

Cooking Instructions:

1. Spread 1 tbsp of peanut butter on each rice cake.
2. Top each with banana slices.
3. Serve immediately.

Cook Tips:

- Use almond butter as a variation or add a sprinkle of cinnamon for extra flavor.
- These can be prepped in advance but should be eaten shortly after assembly to keep the rice cakes crunchy.

Nutritional Value (per serving):

- Calories: 220
- Protein: 6g
- Carbohydrates: 25g
- Fat: 12g
- Fiber: 4g

Low-FODMAP Trail Mix (No Raisins)

Ingredients:

- 1/2 cup almonds
- 1/2 cup walnuts
- 1/4 cup pumpkin seeds
- 1/4 cup sunflower seeds
- 1/4 cup dried cranberries (unsweetened)
- 1/4 cup shredded coconut (unsweetened)

Cooking Instructions:

1. In a bowl, combine the almonds, walnuts, pumpkin seeds, sunflower seeds, cranberries, and shredded coconut.
2. Store in an airtight container for snacking throughout the week.

Cook Tips:

- Add some Low-FODMAP dark chocolate chips for a sweet twist.
- Portion out the mix into snack-size containers for easy grab-and-go snacks.

Nutritional Value (per serving):

- Calories: 250
- Protein: 8g
- Carbohydrates: 12g
- Fat: 20g
- Fiber: 5g

Lactose-Free Yogurt with Raspberries

Ingredients:

- 1 cup lactose-free plain yogurt
- 1/4 cup fresh raspberries
- 1 tsp maple syrup or honey (optional)

Cooking Instructions:

1. Scoop the yogurt into a bowl and top with raspberries.
2. Drizzle with maple syrup or honey if desired.

3. Serve immediately.

Cook Tips:

- You can substitute with blueberries or strawberries for variety.
- Add chia seeds or ground flaxseeds for an extra boost of fiber.

Nutritional Value (per serving):

- Calories: 150
- Protein: 8g
- Carbohydrates: 15g
- Fat: 7g
- Fiber: 4g

Kale Chips with Olive Oil and Sea Salt

Ingredients:

- 1 bunch kale, stems removed and leaves torn into bite-sized pieces
- 1 tbsp olive oil
- 1/2 tsp sea salt

Cooking Instructions:

1. Preheat your oven to 300°F (150°C) and line a baking sheet with parchment paper.
2. Toss the kale pieces with olive oil and sea salt.
3. Spread the kale on the baking sheet in a single layer.
4. Bake for 15-20 minutes, flipping halfway through, until crispy.
5. Let cool before serving.

Cook Tips:

- Keep an eye on the kale as it bakes to prevent burning.

- Sprinkle with nutritional yeast for a cheesy flavor without dairy.

Nutritional Value (per serving):

- Calories: 80
- Protein: 3g
- Carbohydrates: 7g
- Fat: 5g
- Fiber: 2g

Oat and Almond Energy Balls

Ingredients:

- 1 cup gluten-free oats
- 1/2 cup almond butter
- 1/4 cup shredded coconut (unsweetened)
- 1/4 cup maple syrup
- 1 tbsp chia seeds

Cooking Instructions:

1. In a large bowl, mix the oats, almond butter, shredded coconut, maple syrup, and chia seeds until well combined.
2. Roll the mixture into small balls and place them on a baking sheet lined with parchment paper.
3. Refrigerate for at least 30 minutes to set.
4. Store in an airtight container in the fridge.

Cook Tips:

- Add Low-FODMAP chocolate chips or dried cranberries for added flavor.
- These can be frozen for up to a month for easy snacking later.

Nutritional Value (per serving):

- Calories: 180
- Protein: 5g
- Carbohydrates: 20g
- Fat: 9g
- Fiber: 4g

Coconut Macaroons

Ingredients:

- 2 cups shredded coconut (unsweetened)
- 2 egg whites
- 1/4 cup maple syrup
- 1 tsp vanilla extract

Cooking Instructions:

1. Preheat your oven to 325°F (160°C) and line a baking sheet with parchment paper.
2. In a bowl, mix the shredded coconut, egg whites, maple syrup, and vanilla extract until combined.
3. Drop spoonfuls of the mixture onto the baking sheet.
4. Bake for 15-18 minutes, until the edges are golden brown.
5. Let cool before serving.

Cook Tips:

- Dip the bottoms of the macaroons in melted dark chocolate for an indulgent treat.
- These store well in an airtight container for up to a week.

Nutritional Value (per serving):

- Calories: 120
- Protein: 2g
- Carbohydrates: 12g
- Fat: 8g
- Fiber: 3g

Cucumber and Turkey Roll-Ups

Ingredients:

- 1 large cucumber, sliced into long strips
- 4 slices deli turkey (Low-FODMAP certified)
- 2 tbsp lactose-free cream cheese
- 1 tbsp Dijon mustard

Cooking Instructions:

1. Spread a thin layer of lactose-free cream cheese and Dijon mustard onto each turkey slice.
2. Place a cucumber strip on top of each slice and roll up tightly.
3. Secure with a toothpick and serve immediately.

Cook Tips:

- You can add a slice of avocado or fresh herbs for extra flavor.
- These can be prepped in advance and stored in the fridge for up to a day.

Nutritional Value (per serving):

- Calories: 110
- Protein: 10g
- Carbohydrates: 4g

- Fat: 6g
- Fiber: 1g

Gluten-Free Crackers with Goat Cheese

Ingredients:

- 10 gluten-free crackers
- 2 oz goat cheese (lactose-free)
- 1 tbsp fresh herbs (such as parsley or chives)

Cooking Instructions:

1. Spread a small amount of goat cheese onto each gluten-free cracker.
2. Sprinkle with fresh herbs and serve immediately.

Cook Tips:

- Use different herbs like thyme or basil to switch up the flavor.
- This snack pairs well with fresh cucumber or carrot slices.

Nutritional Value (per serving):

- Calories: 150
- Protein: 6g
- Carbohydrates: 18g
- Fat: 7g
- Fiber: 2g

Apple Slices with Almond Butter

Ingredients:

- 1 medium apple, sliced
- 2 tbsp almond butter

Cooking Instructions:

1. Serve apple slices with a small bowl of almond butter for dipping.

Cook Tips:

- Sprinkle the apple slices with a pinch of cinnamon for extra flavor.
- Use Low-FODMAP peanut butter as an alternative to almond butter.

Nutritional Value (per serving):

- Calories: 190
- Protein: 4g
- Carbohydrates: 26g
- Fat: 9g
- Fiber: 5g

Hard-Boiled Eggs with Sea Salt

Ingredients:

- 4 large eggs
- Sea salt to taste

Cooking Instructions:

1. Place the eggs in a saucepan and cover them with cold water.
2. Bring to a boil, then remove from heat and cover. Let sit for 10-12 minutes.
3. Drain and cool the eggs in cold water. Peel and serve with a sprinkle of sea salt.

Cook Tips:

- Store hard-boiled eggs in the fridge for up to one week for quick snacks.
- Serve with Low-FODMAP veggies like cucumber or carrot sticks for a complete snack.

Nutritional Value (per serving):

- Calories: 70
- Protein: 6g
- Carbohydrates: 1g
- Fat: 5g
- Fiber: 0g

Chia Seed Pudding with Strawberries

Ingredients:

- 1/4 cup chia seeds
- 1 cup lactose-free milk or almond milk
- 1 tsp vanilla extract
- 1 tbsp maple syrup
- 1/4 cup fresh strawberries, sliced

Cooking Instructions:

1. In a bowl, mix together the chia seeds, milk, vanilla extract, and maple syrup.
2. Let sit for 5 minutes, then stir again to prevent clumping.
3. Cover and refrigerate for at least 2 hours or overnight until the mixture thickens.
4. Serve topped with fresh strawberries.

Cook Tips:

- Add a sprinkle of Low-FODMAP granola for a crunchy topping.
- This pudding can be made in advance and stored in the fridge for up to 3 days.

Nutritional Value (per serving):

- Calories: 200
- Protein: 6g
- Carbohydrates: 20g
- Fat: 10g
- Fiber: 8g

Zucchini Fritters

Ingredients:

- 2 medium zucchinis, grated
- 1 egg
- 1/4 cup gluten-free flour
- 1/4 cup Parmesan cheese, grated
- 1 tbsp garlic-infused oil
- Salt and pepper to taste

Cooking Instructions:

1. Squeeze out the excess moisture from the grated zucchini using a kitchen towel.
2. In a bowl, mix together the zucchini, egg, flour, Parmesan cheese, salt, and pepper.
3. Heat the garlic-infused oil in a skillet over medium heat.
4. Scoop spoonfuls of the zucchini mixture into the skillet and flatten them into fritters. Cook for 3-4 minutes on each side until golden brown.
5. Serve warm.

Cook Tips:

- You can serve the fritters with a side of lactose-free sour cream or Low-FODMAP salsa.

- Make extra fritters and freeze them for quick snacks or meals later.

Nutritional Value (per serving):

- Calories: 150
- Protein: 6g
- Carbohydrates: 12g
- Fat: 8g
- Fiber: 3g

Chapter 5: Desserts to Satisfy Your Sweet Tooth

Low-FODMAP Chocolate Brownies

Ingredients:

- 1/2 cup lactose-free butter or coconut oil
- 1 cup dark chocolate (Low-FODMAP, 70% or higher)
- 3/4 cup gluten-free all-purpose flour
- 1/2 cup cocoa powder
- 1 cup sugar
- 3 large eggs
- 1 tsp vanilla extract
- A pinch of salt

Cooking Instructions:

1. Preheat your oven to 350°F (175°C) and line an 8x8-inch baking pan with parchment paper.
2. Melt the butter and dark chocolate in a double boiler or microwave, stirring until smooth. Set aside to cool slightly.
3. In a separate bowl, whisk together the sugar, eggs, and vanilla extract.
4. Stir in the melted chocolate mixture until well combined.
5. Sift in the gluten-free flour, cocoa powder, and salt, and fold gently until the batter is smooth.
6. Pour the batter into the prepared baking pan and bake for 20-25 minutes or until a toothpick inserted into the center comes out clean.
7. Let the brownies cool completely before cutting into squares.

Cook Tips:

- For extra richness, fold in some Low-FODMAP chocolate chips or nuts.

- Store leftovers in an airtight container for up to 5 days.

Nutritional Value (per serving):

- Calories: 210
- Protein: 4g
- Carbohydrates: 26g
- Fat: 12g
- Fiber: 3g

Lemon Coconut Macaroons

Ingredients:

- 2 cups shredded coconut (unsweetened)
- 2 egg whites
- 1/4 cup maple syrup or honey
- 1 tsp lemon zest
- 1 tsp vanilla extract

Cooking Instructions:

1. Preheat your oven to 325°F (160°C) and line a baking sheet with parchment paper.
2. In a bowl, whisk the egg whites until frothy, then stir in the maple syrup, vanilla extract, and lemon zest.
3. Fold in the shredded coconut until evenly coated.
4. Drop spoonfuls of the mixture onto the baking sheet and shape them into small mounds.
5. Bake for 15-18 minutes, until the edges are golden.
6. Let the macaroons cool on the baking sheet for 10 minutes before transferring them to a wire rack to cool completely.

Cook Tips:

- For a fancy touch, dip the bottoms of the macaroons in melted Low-FODMAP dark chocolate.
- These can be stored in an airtight container for up to a week.

Nutritional Value (per serving):

- Calories: 110
- Protein: 2g
- Carbohydrates: 12g
- Fat: 7g
- Fiber: 3g

Lactose-Free Vanilla Ice Cream

Ingredients:

- 2 cups lactose-free heavy cream
- 1 cup lactose-free milk
- 1/2 cup sugar
- 1 tbsp vanilla extract
- A pinch of salt

Cooking Instructions:

1. In a saucepan, heat the lactose-free milk and sugar over medium heat, stirring until the sugar dissolves. Remove from heat.
2. Stir in the lactose-free heavy cream, vanilla extract, and a pinch of salt.
3. Pour the mixture into an ice cream maker and churn according to the manufacturer's instructions.
4. Once churned, transfer the ice cream to a container and freeze for at least 4 hours before serving.

Cook Tips:

- For extra flavor, stir in Low-FODMAP add-ins like chopped nuts or chocolate chips before freezing.
- If you don't have an ice cream maker, you can pour the mixture into a shallow dish and freeze, stirring every 30 minutes until smooth.

Nutritional Value (per serving):

- Calories: 200
- Protein: 2g
- Carbohydrates: 20g
- Fat: 12g
- Fiber: 0g

Almond Flour Chocolate Chip Cookies

Ingredients:

- 2 cups almond flour
- 1/4 cup coconut oil, melted
- 1/4 cup maple syrup
- 1 egg
- 1 tsp vanilla extract
- 1/2 tsp baking soda
- 1/2 cup Low-FODMAP dark chocolate chips
- A pinch of salt

Cooking Instructions:

1. Preheat your oven to 350°F (175°C) and line a baking sheet with parchment paper.

2. In a bowl, mix together the melted coconut oil, maple syrup, egg, and vanilla extract.

3. Add the almond flour, baking soda, and salt, and stir until a dough forms.

4. Fold in the Low-FODMAP chocolate chips.

5. Drop spoonfuls of dough onto the baking sheet and gently flatten each one.

6. Bake for 10-12 minutes, until the edges are golden.

7. Let the cookies cool on the baking sheet for 5 minutes before transferring them to a wire rack.

Cook Tips:

- These cookies can be stored in an airtight container for up to a week.
- You can also add Low-FODMAP nuts or seeds for a crunchy twist.

Nutritional Value (per serving):

- Calories: 160
- Protein: 4g
- Carbohydrates: 10g
- Fat: 12g
- Fiber: 3g

Gluten-Free Blueberry Muffins

Ingredients:

- 1 1/2 cups gluten-free all-purpose flour
- 1/2 cup lactose-free yogurt
- 1/4 cup coconut oil, melted
- 2 eggs
- 1/2 cup sugar
- 1 tsp vanilla extract
- 1 tsp baking powder

- 1/2 tsp baking soda
- 1 cup fresh or frozen blueberries

Cooking Instructions:

1. Preheat your oven to 350°F (175°C) and line a muffin tin with paper liners.
2. In a bowl, whisk together the lactose-free yogurt, melted coconut oil, eggs, sugar, and vanilla extract.
3. In a separate bowl, combine the gluten-free flour, baking powder, and baking soda.
4. Add the dry ingredients to the wet mixture and stir until just combined.
5. Fold in the blueberries.
6. Divide the batter evenly among the muffin cups and bake for 18-20 minutes, until a toothpick inserted into the center comes out clean.
7. Let the muffins cool in the tin for 5 minutes before transferring them to a wire rack.

Cook Tips:

- For an extra burst of flavor, add a pinch of lemon zest to the batter.
- These muffins freeze well, making them great for meal prep.

Nutritional Value (per serving):

- Calories: 180
- Protein: 5g
- Carbohydrates: 25g
- Fat: 8g
- Fiber: 3g

Pumpkin Pie (Low-FODMAP Crust)

Ingredients:

For the Crust:

- 1 1/4 cups gluten-free all-purpose flour
- 1/2 cup lactose-free butter, chilled and cubed
- 1/4 cup ice water
- 1/2 tsp salt

For the Filling:

- 1 cup canned pumpkin puree
- 1/2 cup lactose-free milk or cream
- 2 eggs
- 1/2 cup maple syrup
- 1 tsp vanilla extract
- 1 tsp ground cinnamon
- 1/2 tsp ground ginger
- 1/4 tsp ground nutmeg
- A pinch of salt

Cooking Instructions:

1. Preheat your oven to 350°F (175°C).
2. To make the crust, combine the gluten-free flour and salt in a bowl. Cut in the chilled butter until the mixture resembles coarse crumbs.
3. Gradually add the ice water, mixing until a dough forms. Press the dough into a pie dish and set aside.
4. In a separate bowl, whisk together the pumpkin puree, lactose-free milk, eggs, maple syrup, vanilla extract, cinnamon, ginger, nutmeg, and salt.
5. Pour the filling into the prepared crust and smooth the top.
6. Bake for 45-50 minutes, or until the filling is set and the crust is golden.

7. Let the pie cool before slicing.

Cook Tips:

- Top the pie with a dollop of lactose-free whipped cream for an extra treat.
- Store leftovers in the fridge for up to 4 days.

Nutritional Value (per serving):

- Calories: 260
- Protein: 4g
- Carbohydrates: 30g
- Fat: 12g
- Fiber: 3g

Banana Bread with Walnuts (Gluten-Free)

Ingredients:

- 2 ripe bananas
- 2 eggs
- 1/4 cup coconut oil, melted
- 1/4 cup maple syrup
- 1 tsp vanilla extract
- 1 1/2 cups gluten-free all-purpose flour
- 1 tsp baking soda
- 1/2 cup chopped walnuts
- A pinch of salt

Cooking Instructions:

1. Preheat your oven to 350°F (175°C) and grease a loaf pan.
2. In a bowl, mash the bananas until smooth. Stir in the eggs, melted coconut oil, maple syrup, and vanilla extract.

3. In another bowl, whisk together the gluten-free flour, baking soda, and salt.

4. Gradually add the dry ingredients to the wet mixture and stir until just combined.

5. Fold in the chopped walnuts.

6. Pour the batter into the prepared loaf pan and bake for 50-60 minutes, or until a toothpick inserted into the center comes out clean.

7. Let the bread cool in the pan for 10 minutes before transferring it to a wire rack.

Cook Tips:

- You can add Low-FODMAP chocolate chips for a sweeter twist.
- This banana bread freezes well for later use.

Nutritional Value (per serving):

- Calories: 200
- Protein: 5g
- Carbohydrates: 25g
- Fat: 10g
- Fiber: 3g

Coconut Rice Pudding with Mango

Ingredients:

- 1/2 cup jasmine rice
- 1 1/2 cups lactose-free coconut milk
- 1/4 cup sugar
- 1 tsp vanilla extract
- 1/2 cup fresh mango, diced

Cooking Instructions:

1. In a saucepan, combine the jasmine rice, lactose-free coconut milk, and sugar. Bring to a boil, then reduce to a simmer and cook for 15-20 minutes, stirring occasionally, until the rice is tender and the mixture thickens.
2. Stir in the vanilla extract and remove from heat.
3. Divide the rice pudding into bowls and top with fresh diced mango.
4. Serve warm or chilled.

Cook Tips:

- For a creamier pudding, stir in more coconut milk as it cools.
- This rice pudding can be stored in the fridge for up to 3 days.

Nutritional Value (per serving):

- Calories: 180
- Protein: 3g
- Carbohydrates: 35g
- Fat: 4g
- Fiber: 2g

Low-FODMAP Apple Crisp

Ingredients:

- 4 medium apples (peeled, cored, and sliced)
- 1/2 cup gluten-free oats
- 1/4 cup almond flour
- 1/4 cup coconut oil (melted)
- 1/4 cup maple syrup
- 1 tsp cinnamon
- 1/4 tsp nutmeg
- A pinch of salt

Cooking Instructions:

1. Preheat your oven to 350°F (175°C) and grease a baking dish.
2. In a bowl, toss the apple slices with 1 tbsp maple syrup and a pinch of cinnamon. Spread them evenly in the baking dish.
3. In another bowl, combine the oats, almond flour, melted coconut oil, maple syrup, cinnamon, nutmeg, and salt. Stir until a crumbly mixture forms.
4. Sprinkle the oat mixture over the apples, covering them evenly.
5. Bake for 30-35 minutes, or until the apples are tender and the topping is golden brown.
6. Let the crisp cool for a few minutes before serving.

Cook Tips:

- Serve with a scoop of lactose-free vanilla ice cream for a decadent dessert.
- You can use a combination of apples and pears for variety.

Nutritional Value (per serving):

- Calories: 220
- Protein: 3g
- Carbohydrates: 35g
- Fat: 10g
- Fiber: 5g

Peanut Butter Fudge (Lactose-Free)

Ingredients:

- 1 cup natural peanut butter (unsweetened)
- 1/4 cup coconut oil (melted)
- 1/4 cup maple syrup
- 1 tsp vanilla extract

- A pinch of salt

Cooking Instructions:

1. Line a small square baking dish with parchment paper.
2. In a bowl, mix together the peanut butter, melted coconut oil, maple syrup, vanilla extract, and salt until smooth.
3. Pour the mixture into the prepared baking dish and spread it out evenly.
4. Freeze for 2-3 hours until firm.
5. Once set, cut the fudge into small squares and serve.

Cook Tips:

- Store the fudge in the freezer for up to two weeks.
- You can swirl in Low-FODMAP dark chocolate for a richer flavor.

Nutritional Value (per serving):

- Calories: 180
- Protein: 4g
- Carbohydrates: 10g
- Fat: 14g
- Fiber: 2g

Lemon Bars with Almond Crust

Ingredients:

For the Crust:

- 1 cup almond flour
- 2 tbsp coconut oil (melted)
- 2 tbsp maple syrup

For the Lemon Filling:

- 3 large eggs
- 1/2 cup lemon juice (freshly squeezed)
- 1/4 cup maple syrup
- 1 tbsp lemon zest
- 1 tbsp gluten-free flour
- A pinch of salt

Cooking Instructions:

1. Preheat your oven to 350°F (175°C) and line an 8x8-inch baking pan with parchment paper.
2. In a bowl, mix the almond flour, melted coconut oil, and maple syrup to form a dough. Press it evenly into the bottom of the prepared pan.
3. Bake the crust for 10-12 minutes, or until lightly golden.
4. In a separate bowl, whisk together the eggs, lemon juice, maple syrup, lemon zest, gluten-free flour, and salt.
5. Pour the lemon filling over the baked crust and return to the oven. Bake for 20-25 minutes, or until the filling is set.
6. Let the bars cool completely before slicing.

Cook Tips:

- Dust the tops of the bars with a little powdered sugar for presentation.
- Store the bars in the fridge for up to 5 days.

Nutritional Value (per serving):

- Calories: 160
- Protein: 4g
- Carbohydrates: 15g
- Fat: 10g
- Fiber: 2g

Gluten-Free Carrot Cake

Ingredients:

For the Cake:

- 1 1/2 cups gluten-free all-purpose flour
- 1/2 cup coconut oil (melted)
- 3/4 cup brown sugar
- 2 eggs
- 1 cup grated carrots
- 1/4 cup chopped walnuts
- 1 tsp cinnamon
- 1 tsp baking powder
- 1/2 tsp baking soda
- A pinch of salt

For the Frosting:

- 1/2 cup lactose-free cream cheese
- 1/4 cup powdered sugar
- 1 tsp vanilla extract

Cooking Instructions:

1. Preheat your oven to 350°F (175°C) and grease a 9-inch round cake pan.
2. In a bowl, whisk together the melted coconut oil, brown sugar, and eggs until smooth.
3. In another bowl, combine the gluten-free flour, cinnamon, baking powder, baking soda, and salt.
4. Gradually add the dry ingredients to the wet mixture, stirring until just combined. Fold in the grated carrots and chopped walnuts.

5. Pour the batter into the prepared cake pan and bake for 30-35 minutes, or until a toothpick inserted into the center comes out clean.

6. Let the cake cool completely before frosting.

7. To make the frosting, beat together the lactose-free cream cheese, powdered sugar, and vanilla extract until smooth. Spread the frosting over the cooled cake.

Cook Tips:

- You can make cupcakes instead of a whole cake by dividing the batter into a muffin tin.
- For extra flavor, add a sprinkle of shredded coconut on top of the frosting.

Nutritional Value (per serving):

- Calories: 250
- Protein: 5g
- Carbohydrates: 30g
- Fat: 12g
- Fiber: 3g

Raspberry Sorbet

Ingredients:

- 2 cups fresh or frozen raspberries
- 1/4 cup maple syrup
- 1/2 cup water
- 1 tbsp lemon juice

Cooking Instructions:

1. In a blender or food processor, combine the raspberries, maple syrup, water, and lemon juice. Blend until smooth.

2. Strain the mixture through a fine-mesh sieve to remove the seeds.

3. Pour the raspberry mixture into an ice cream maker and churn according to the manufacturer's instructions.

4. Once churned, transfer the sorbet to a container and freeze for at least 2 hours before serving.

Cook Tips:

- If you don't have an ice cream maker, pour the mixture into a shallow dish and freeze, stirring every 30 minutes until smooth.
- Serve with fresh mint leaves or a few extra raspberries for garnish.

Nutritional Value (per serving):

- Calories: 100
- Protein: 1g
- Carbohydrates: 25g
- Fat: 0g
- Fiber: 6g

Vanilla Chia Seed Pudding

Ingredients:

- 1/4 cup chia seeds
- 1 cup lactose-free milk or almond milk
- 1 tsp vanilla extract
- 1 tbsp maple syrup
- 1/4 cup fresh berries (for topping)

Cooking Instructions:

1. In a bowl, mix together the chia seeds, milk, vanilla extract, and maple syrup.

2. Let the mixture sit for 5 minutes, then stir again to prevent clumping.

3. Cover and refrigerate for at least 2 hours or overnight until the mixture thickens into a pudding-like consistency.

4. Serve topped with fresh berries.

Cook Tips:

- Add a sprinkle of cinnamon or shredded coconut for extra flavor.
- You can store the pudding in the fridge for up to 3 days for easy make-ahead breakfasts.

Nutritional Value (per serving):

- Calories: 200
- Protein: 6g
- Carbohydrates: 20g
- Fat: 10g
- Fiber: 8g

Baked Pears with Cinnamon and Honey

Ingredients:

- 4 ripe pears, halved and cored
- 2 tbsp honey
- 1 tsp cinnamon
- 1/4 cup chopped walnuts (optional)

Cooking Instructions:

1. Preheat your oven to 350°F (175°C) and line a baking dish with parchment paper.
2. Place the pear halves in the baking dish, cut side up.
3. Drizzle the pears with honey and sprinkle with cinnamon.
4. Bake for 20-25 minutes, or until the pears are tender and slightly caramelized.
5. Remove from the oven and sprinkle with chopped walnuts, if using. Serve warm.

Cook Tips:

- Pair the baked pears with a scoop of lactose-free vanilla ice cream or a dollop of whipped cream.
- For a variation, add a splash of vanilla extract or lemon juice before baking.

Nutritional Value (per serving):

- Calories: 150
- Protein: 2g
- Carbohydrates: 30g
- Fat: 4g
- Fiber: 5g

Chapter 6: Drinks and Smoothies for a Gut-Friendly Boost

Green Smoothie with Spinach and Banana

Ingredients:

- 1/2 cup fresh spinach
- 1/2 unripe banana (green)
- 1/2 cup lactose-free yogurt or almond milk
- 1 tbsp chia seeds
- 1/4 cup water
- 1 tbsp maple syrup (optional)

Cooking Instructions:

1. In a blender, combine the spinach, banana, lactose-free yogurt or almond milk, chia seeds, water, and maple syrup.
2. Blend until smooth and creamy.
3. Serve immediately.

Cook Tips:

- Use frozen spinach or banana for a thicker, colder smoothie.
- Add ice cubes if you prefer a chilled drink.

Nutritional Value (per serving):

- Calories: 160
- Protein: 5g
- Carbohydrates: 25g
- Fat: 4g
- Fiber: 5g

Low-FODMAP Blueberry Almond Smoothie

Ingredients:

- 1/2 cup fresh or frozen blueberries
- 1/2 cup almond milk (unsweetened)
- 1 tbsp almond butter
- 1 tbsp chia seeds
- 1/2 tsp vanilla extract

Cooking Instructions:

1. Combine the blueberries, almond milk, almond butter, chia seeds, and vanilla extract in a blender.
2. Blend until smooth and creamy.
3. Pour into a glass and enjoy!

Cook Tips:

- You can substitute the almond butter with peanut butter for a different flavor.
- For a thicker smoothie, add a handful of ice cubes before blending.

Nutritional Value (per serving):

- Calories: 200
- Protein: 6g
- Carbohydrates: 20g
- Fat: 12g
- Fiber: 6g

Ginger and Lemon Infused Water

Ingredients:

- 1-inch piece fresh ginger, sliced
- 1/2 lemon, sliced
- 4 cups water

Cooking Instructions:

1. Add the ginger and lemon slices to a pitcher of water.
2. Let the water infuse in the fridge for at least 1-2 hours before serving.
3. Serve chilled.

Cook Tips:

- For a stronger flavor, leave the water to infuse overnight.
- Add ice cubes and mint leaves for extra freshness.

Nutritional Value (per serving):

- Calories: 5
- Protein: 0g
- Carbohydrates: 1g
- Fat: 0g
- Fiber: 0g

Lactose-Free Chai Latte

Ingredients:

- 1 cup lactose-free milk
- 1 chai tea bag
- 1 tsp maple syrup or honey

- 1/2 tsp ground cinnamon
- 1/4 tsp ground ginger
- A pinch of ground cloves

Cooking Instructions:

1. Heat the lactose-free milk in a saucepan over medium heat until warm.
2. Add the chai tea bag and steep for 5-7 minutes.
3. Stir in the maple syrup or honey, cinnamon, ginger, and cloves.
4. Remove the tea bag and whisk the milk until frothy.
5. Pour into a mug and serve warm.

Cook Tips:

- For a creamier latte, use lactose-free cream instead of milk.
- You can serve this latte over ice for a refreshing iced chai version.

Nutritional Value (per serving):

- Calories: 120
- Protein: 6g
- Carbohydrates: 15g
- Fat: 4g
- Fiber: 1g

FODMAP-Friendly Iced Coffee

Ingredients:

- 1/2 cup brewed coffee (chilled)
- 1/2 cup lactose-free milk or almond milk
- 1 tbsp maple syrup or stevia (optional)
- Ice cubes

Cooking Instructions:

1. Fill a glass with ice cubes.
2. Pour the chilled coffee over the ice.
3. Add lactose-free milk or almond milk and stir in maple syrup or stevia if desired.
4. Serve immediately.

Cook Tips:

- Brew your coffee the night before and chill it in the fridge for a quicker preparation.
- For an extra treat, add a splash of vanilla extract or a sprinkle of cinnamon.

Nutritional Value (per serving):

- Calories: 60
- Protein: 2g
- Carbohydrates: 8g
- Fat: 2g
- Fiber: 0g

Herbal Digestive Tea Blend

Ingredients:

- 1 tbsp dried peppermint leaves
- 1 tbsp dried chamomile flowers
- 1 tsp dried fennel seeds
- 4 cups water

Cooking Instructions:

1. In a teapot, combine the peppermint leaves, chamomile flowers, and fennel seeds.

2. Pour boiling water over the herbs and steep for 10 minutes.

3. Strain the tea into cups and serve warm.

Cook Tips:

- Sweeten with a little honey if desired.
- This tea can also be served chilled over ice for a refreshing iced tea.

Nutritional Value (per serving):

- Calories: 0
- Protein: 0g
- Carbohydrates: 0g
- Fat: 0g
- Fiber: 0g

Low-FODMAP Electrolyte Drink

Ingredients:

- 1 cup coconut water
- 1/2 cup water
- 1/4 cup fresh orange juice
- 1 tbsp lemon juice
- A pinch of salt

Cooking Instructions:

1. In a glass, mix the coconut water, water, orange juice, lemon juice, and a pinch of salt.

2. Stir well and serve chilled or over ice.

Cook Tips:

- Add a few mint leaves for extra flavor.
- This drink is perfect for hydration after exercise.

Nutritional Value (per serving):

- Calories: 60
- Protein: 1g
- Carbohydrates: 15g
- Fat: 0g
- Fiber: 1g

Pineapple and Mint Smoothie

Ingredients:

- 1/2 cup fresh or frozen pineapple chunks
- 1/4 cup lactose-free yogurt
- 1/4 cup coconut water
- 4-5 fresh mint leaves
- Ice cubes (optional)

Cooking Instructions:

1. Combine the pineapple chunks, lactose-free yogurt, coconut water, and mint leaves in a blender.
2. Blend until smooth and creamy.
3. Serve immediately, garnished with extra mint leaves if desired.

Cook Tips:

- For a creamier smoothie, add a little more yogurt or a frozen banana.
- You can also use coconut milk instead of coconut water for a richer flavor.

Nutritional Value (per serving):

- Calories: 150
- Protein: 4g
- Carbohydrates: 30g
- Fat: 3g
- Fiber: 2g

Strawberry Lemonade (Low-FODMAP)

Ingredients:

- 1 cup fresh strawberries, hulled
- 1/4 cup lemon juice (freshly squeezed)
- 2 cups water
- 2 tbsp maple syrup or stevia
- Ice cubes

Cooking Instructions:

1. Blend the strawberries with 1 cup of water until smooth.
2. Strain the strawberry puree to remove the seeds.
3. In a pitcher, mix the strained strawberry puree with the remaining water, lemon juice, and maple syrup or stevia.
4. Stir well and serve over ice.

Cook Tips:

- Garnish with lemon slices and fresh mint for extra freshness.
- Adjust the sweetness to your preference by adding more or less maple syrup or stevia.

Nutritional Value (per serving):

- Calories: 50
- Protein: 1g
- Carbohydrates: 12g
- Fat: 0g
- Fiber: 2g

Lactose-Free Hot Chocolate

Ingredients:

- 1 cup lactose-free milk
- 2 tbsp unsweetened cocoa powder
- 1 tbsp maple syrup or stevia
- 1/2 tsp vanilla extract

Cooking Instructions:

1. Heat the lactose-free milk in a saucepan over medium heat until warm.
2. Whisk in the cocoa powder, maple syrup, and vanilla extract until smooth.
3. Pour into a mug and serve warm.

Cook Tips:

- Add a pinch of cinnamon or nutmeg for extra flavor.
- Top with lactose-free whipped cream or marshmallows for an indulgent treat.

Nutritional Value (per serving):

- Calories: 120
- Protein: 6g
- Carbohydrates: 15g
- Fat: 4g

- Fiber: 2g

Cucumber and Lime Detox Water

Ingredients:

- 1/2 cucumber, thinly sliced
- 1 lime, thinly sliced
- 4 cups water

Cooking Instructions:

1. In a pitcher, combine the cucumber and lime slices.
2. Pour the water over the cucumber and lime, and let it infuse in the fridge for at least 1-2 hours before serving.
3. Serve chilled.

Cook Tips:

- Add a few mint leaves or basil for a refreshing twist.
- This detox water is perfect for staying hydrated throughout the day.

Nutritional Value (per serving):

- Calories: 5
- Protein: 0g
- Carbohydrates: 1g
- Fat: 0g
- Fiber: 0g

Coconut Water with Berries

Ingredients:

- 1 cup coconut water
- 1/4 cup fresh raspberries or blueberries
- Ice cubes

Cooking Instructions:

1. In a glass, add the fresh berries and coconut water.
2. Stir well and serve over ice.

Cook Tips:

- Muddle the berries before adding the coconut water for a more intense flavor.
- You can add a squeeze of lime juice for extra tang.

Nutritional Value (per serving):

- Calories: 60
- Protein: 1g
- Carbohydrates: 15g
- Fat: 0g
- Fiber: 2g

Anti-Inflammatory Turmeric Tea

Ingredients:

- 1 cup lactose-free milk or almond milk
- 1/2 tsp ground turmeric
- 1/4 tsp ground ginger
- 1 tbsp maple syrup or honey

- A pinch of black pepper

Cooking Instructions:

1. In a small saucepan, heat the lactose-free milk or almond milk over medium heat.
2. Stir in the turmeric, ginger, maple syrup, and black pepper.
3. Whisk until well combined and heated through.
4. Serve warm.

Cook Tips:

- Add a pinch of cinnamon for extra warmth and flavor.
- This tea can also be served cold over ice.

Nutritional Value (per serving):

- Calories: 120
- Protein: 2g
- Carbohydrates: 20g
- Fat: 4g
- Fiber: 1g

Raspberry and Basil Iced Tea

Ingredients:

- 2 cups water
- 1/2 cup fresh raspberries
- 4-5 fresh basil leaves
- 1 green tea bag
- 1 tbsp maple syrup or honey (optional)

Cooking Instructions:

1. Boil the water and steep the green tea bag for 5 minutes.
2. Muddle the raspberries and basil leaves in a glass.
3. Pour the brewed green tea over the muddled raspberries and basil.
4. Add ice cubes and stir well. Sweeten with maple syrup or honey if desired.

Cook Tips:

- Garnish with extra raspberries and basil leaves for a beautiful presentation.
- This tea can be made in advance and stored in the fridge for up to 2 days.

Nutritional Value (per serving):

- Calories: 30
- Protein: 0g
- Carbohydrates: 8g
- Fat: 0g
- Fiber: 2g

Lactose-Free Vanilla Milkshake

Ingredients:

- 1 cup lactose-free vanilla ice cream
- 1/2 cup lactose-free milk or almond milk
- 1/2 tsp vanilla extract
- Ice cubes (optional)

Cooking Instructions:

1. Combine the lactose-free vanilla ice cream, lactose-free milk, and vanilla extract in a blender.
2. Blend until smooth and creamy.

3. Serve immediately in a chilled glass.

Cook Tips:

- Add Low-FODMAP chocolate chips or a swirl of Low-FODMAP caramel sauce for a fun twist.
- You can also make a thicker shake by adding more ice cream or ice cubes.

Nutritional Value (per serving):

- Calories: 200
- Protein: 4g
- Carbohydrates: 30g
- Fat: 8g
- Fiber: 0g

Conclusion

As you reach the conclusion of your journey through the Low-FODMAP diet, it's essential to reflect on how far you've come and where you're headed. The initial challenges of adjusting to a new way of eating may have seemed daunting, but with time, dedication, and experimentation, you've gained a deeper understanding of your body and its needs. The ultimate goal is not to follow a restrictive diet forever but to create a sustainable and balanced lifestyle that minimizes discomfort and maximizes your enjoyment of food.

The **gradual reintroduction of foods** is the next critical step in your long-term success. The Low-FODMAP diet isn't about permanently eliminating all high-FODMAP foods but about identifying which specific foods trigger your symptoms. By reintroducing these foods slowly and methodically, you can discover your personal tolerances. Some foods may be reintroduced without issue, while others may need to remain limited. This process will empower you to make informed choices that allow you to enjoy a varied diet without triggering unwanted symptoms. Keep a food diary during this phase to track your reactions and ensure that you're reintroducing foods one at a time for accurate results.

Managing IBS symptoms long-term requires mindfulness and patience. There will be times when symptoms flare up, even when you feel you're doing everything right. Stress, travel, or an unintentional slip-up can all contribute to these moments. The key is to stay calm, return to the basics of the Low-FODMAP diet during flare-ups, and remember that you now have the tools to regain control over your digestive health. By staying flexible and open to adjustments, you'll be able to manage symptoms more effectively and minimize their impact on your daily life.

The importance of **continuing to experiment with new recipes** cannot be overstated. Just because you've found a routine that works doesn't mean you should stop exploring new foods and meal ideas. Variety is essential for both nutrition and enjoyment. Over time, you'll likely discover new Low-FODMAP recipes that excite your taste buds and keep your meals interesting. Don't be afraid to experiment with different flavor combinations, cooking methods, and ingredients. You've already proven to yourself that there's a world of delicious, IBS-friendly meals out there, so keep expanding your culinary horizons.

Finally, **maintaining dietary balance** is the cornerstone of long-term success. It's easy to fall into the trap of focusing too much on what you can't eat, but your mindset should now shift to celebrating what you can enjoy. Embrace whole, unprocessed foods that nourish your body, provide energy, and contribute to your overall well-being. Pay attention to portion sizes, hydration, and ensuring that your diet is rich in fiber, vitamins, and minerals from the foods that work well for your digestive system.

The Low-FODMAP diet is more than just a temporary solution for managing IBS symptoms—it's a pathway to understanding your body better and creating a lifestyle that supports your digestive health for the long term. By staying committed to reintroducing foods carefully, managing symptoms with confidence, and keeping your meals varied and balanced, you'll continue to thrive in a way that suits your unique needs. Ultimately, your journey on this diet is about empowerment: knowing that you have the knowledge and resources to live symptom-free while still enjoying the foods that bring you joy.